QUIT SMOKING

Free Yourself from Smoking With No Pain & Hesitation and Start Living a Healthy Life (The Ultimate Guide With Pro Tips)

By CARRIE DRESDEN

Table of Contents

Chapter 1: Introduction

For a non-smoker, it is really easy to get rid of nicotine addiction, but honestly, it is not easy. Nicotine is an active addictive ingredient in cigarettes and its addiction is stronger than alcohol. Nicotine excites pleasure centers in your brain because it is highly addictive. Once nicotine is discontinued, the smoker experiences withdrawal symptoms and increases the desire of a person to smoke again and get rid of withdrawal symptoms.

Typical withdrawal symptoms of nicotine are:
- Aches and discomfort
- Irritability
- Sleep deprivation
- Fatigue
- Headache
- Difficulty in concentration
- Sore throat
- Chest tightness
- Sore tongue and gums

Smoking cessation is difficult, but you can do it with strong determination and will power. If you want to make this journey easy, you should focus on the highly rewarding aspects of smoking cessation. After smoking cessation, the first few weeks will be hardest and after 8 to 12 weeks, you will start feeling more relaxed without smoking. Becoming a non-smoker is really challenging, but this effort is really rewarding.

There are numerous traditional methods that are successfully helping people to quit smoking. These treatments are typically divided into two groups, psychological and behavioral method and anti-smoking medicines. There is no well-defined approach to quitting smoking, but a smoking cessation plan is often designed according to the unique situation of a person.

The basic purpose of this book is to increase your awareness that smoking is destroying your life and you are wasting precious moments of your life for this cruel addiction. By reading this book, you can design a quit plan for you and start a healthy routine.

Chapter 2: Why Is It Important to Quit Smoking?

Smoking cessation can make a big difference to your lifestyle and health. It is never too late to get rid of this habit because you can protect yourself from cancer and other diseases. You can avoid increased risk of early death and enjoy a healthy life with your family. Tobacco contains more than 70,000 chemicals, such as hydrogen cyanide, ammonia, and carbon monoxide. Almost 69 harmful chemicals can cause cancer, such as Acetaldehyde, Aromatic amines, Benzene, Beryllium, Cadmium, Cumene, Chromium, Ethylene Oxide, vinyl chloride are a few of those chemicals that can cause cancer. Tobacco smoke can cause lung cancer, heart disease, respiratory problems, and lots of other diseases. There are a few downsides of smoking that you may not consider:

Health Problems

•   Smoking can fog the mind and you may suffer from memory problems. In the middle age, you may not be able to remember important things and unable to take important decisions of your life.

- Smoking can increase the risk factors for type II diabetes. It may invite different infections by damaging your immune system.

- It can stultify your sex life and a decrease your chances of getting pregnant. You may suffer from erection problems (impotence), fertility problems and various other similar diseases. Women with smoking habits are prone to early menopause.

- Smoking is directly linked to heart diseases, aortic aneurysm (a bulge of arteries in your chest), stroke, COPD (chronic obstructive pulmonary disease), asthma, cataracts, etc.

Passive Smoke

Just because of smoking, you are not only harming yourself, but your family members as well. Passive smoke or secondhand smoke, also known as ETS (environmental tobacco smoke) and a non-smoker is exposed to this smoke. Passive smoke has similar harmful chemicals and it can cause lung cancer, larynx, pharynx and nasal sinus cancer, liver cancer and brain tumor. Second-hand smoke is harmful in numerous ways because it affects the blood vessels and heart; increase the risk of stroke and heart attack, even in non-smokers.

As a smoker, you are not only ruining your health, but affecting the health of people around you. With the passage of time, your body may get an unbearable stink and your children, the even family member will try to avoid you. It can destroy your teeth, nails, and skin color.

Quit smoking is really beneficial for you and after reading hazards of smoking and benefits of smoking cessation, you will really feel motivated to start this beneficial journey.

Chapter 3: Create a Quit Plan to Prepare Yourself

You are planning to quit smoking for a long time because of its risks and expenses. It is really difficult because smoking is a bad habit and you have to motivate yourself. Focus on the benefits of smoking cessation and increase your motivation for this work. Remind yourself that you can do this and you have to do this for you and your family. You may fail numerous attempts, but this time, start with a plan that can keep you organized and maintain your focus on your goal. Keep it in mind that it is difficult to get rid of this addiction. You should have strong will power and determination. There is a sample plan that will help you to make your own plan to quit smoking:

Set a Date to Quite

If you are ready to live a healthy life, decide a date to start your plan. You can select a date within the next 15 days to quit smoking. It will give you sufficient time to prepare and you can think about your date. You should not pick a busy day with lots of stress and temptation to smoke.

Ask for Support of Friends and Family

Your journey to quit smoking can be easy with the support of your friends and family members. You can share your quit plan with others and ask for their help. You should share your reasons for quitting and ask friends and family to keep an eye on your progress.

- You have to identify your smoking triggers and ask your family and friends to help you deal with these triggers. Your family members can help you in the smoke-free activities, such as you can go to a nice restaurant or play a game.

- If any of your friend or family members also smoke, you can ask them to quit this habit with you or, at least, avoid smoking in front of you.

- You will be tempted to smoke, but your friends and family members can help you to avoid smoking.

- It will be good to consult a doctor for any medication and safe replacements to help you quit.

Plan for Challenges

Smoking cessation will be hardest in the initial few weeks and you have to deal with the temptations and uncomfortable feelings, withdrawal symptoms and nicotine cravings. You have to anticipate all these challenges and keep the following things in your mind:

Uncomfortable Feelings

In the first few weeks after smoking cessation, you may feel uncomfortable and crave only one cigarette. It is a withdrawal symptom because your body is not getting nicotine. Nicotine is a harmful chemical in cigarettes to increase your urge to keep smoking.

Other common symptoms of withdrawal are:

- Depressed feelings
- Unable to sleep
- Frustrated, cranky and mad behavior
- Anxious, restless and nervous feelings
- Unable to think clearly

You will be tempted to smoke only one cigarette to get rid of these feelings. Keep it in mind that these are temporary symptoms and you can get rid of them in a few weeks. These can be very powerful, but you have to distract your mind and pay attention to other healthy activities.

Select Your Reasons to Quit

If you want to stay focused and motivated, select a reason for quitting. This should be a part of your quitting plan, such as:

- You are quitting because you want to live a healthy life.
- You want to save money and smell better.
- You want to get rid of a permanent cough.
- Your loved ones are important for you.

Effects of Quit Smoking

After smoking cessation, the nicotine will be out of your system and you can enjoy a better health. Physical withdrawal symptoms will start to fade after two weeks. You can get rid of craving for emotional and habitual triggers between one to two months.

Identify Your Smoking Triggers

You should know your trigger because it will help you to stay in control. At an initial stage, you may want to completely avoid your triggers, but with the passage of time, you may find it easy to handle your triggers. There are a few common triggers, you can select one of them and include in your plan.

Emotional Triggers
- Feeling anxious
- Stressful Feelings

- Feeling lonely
- Feeling down
- Boredom feelings
- Cooling off subsequent to a fight

Habitual Triggers

- Conversation on phone
- Alcohol consumption
- Enjoying Programs on TV
- Driving
- After having sex
- After finishing a meal
- After Tea or Coffee
- Work break

Social Triggers

- Your visit to a bar
- Attending Social Events
- Noticing other smokers

Prepare Yourself to Fight with Craving

It is important to prepare yourself to fight with cravings because these will last only a few minutes. There are some tips that will help you to fight with craving:

Keep Your Hand and Mouth Busy

You can hold a straw in your hand to take a breath through it. Play with a paper ball, clip or coin to keep your hands busy.

Improve Your Mood

- If you want to improve your mood and relieve stress, you can:
- Practice meditation or deep breathing to calm down.
- Push-ups will help you to blow off your inner steam.
- Busy in communication with your friends, family members and counselors.
- Prepare a list of tasks to accomplish during craving hits, such as plan your regular schedule, complete your tasks in hand or reply to your emails.

Treat Yourself

If you smoke for pleasure and relaxation, you can treat yourself with other types of pleasures, such as listen to music, night out with friends or enjoy your favorite desserts with the money that you have saved by leaving cigarettes.

Get Rid of Irritability and Anxious Feelings

NRT (Nicotine Replacement Therapy) can be helpful, such as you can use gum, patches and lozenges to relieve your withdrawal symptoms. You should consult a doctor to find a right NRT for you.

Boost Your Energy

If you smoke for an instant boost in energy, you can increase your energy levels with the following activities:

- Regular exercise and healthy snacks can increase your energy.
- You should enjoy plenty of sleep at night to avoid feeling slow during the day.

Avoid Smoking Reminders

Smoking reminders can make your journey hard and you have to get rid of these reminders in the home, car, and workplace before your quit days. There is a list of smoking reminders and you should add these things to your plan:

- Wash your clothes and cars to get rid of smoke smells and wear clean clothes without any matchstick or cigarette in your clothes.

- Clean your car and throw away all cigarettes and matches.

- Get rid of ashtrays, matches and cigarette butts.

Replace cigarettes, lighters and matchsticks with craving items, such as straws and nicotine gum. You have to make a list of chores and keep in the places instead of ashtrays, lighters, matches and cigarettes. Throw all smoking items almost a night before your quit day and avoid hiding any pack in your freezer or cabinet.

Avoid Tobacco Products

You have to avoid all tobacco products as well because some people quit cigarettes and prefer to chew tobacco. Keep it in mind that tobacco has harmful poisons and chemicals. Stay away from smokeless tobacco, cigars, pipes, hookahs, clove cigarettes, bidi cigarettes, herbal cigarettes and cigarillos because these are equally harmful.

Talk to Pharmacist and Discuss Quit Options

It can be difficult to quit smoking without any professional help. You should talk to your pharmacist or doctor for support options. A qualified doctor can answer your question and advise you to quit smoking easily. You can get NRT therapy, such as nicotine gum, patch or lozenge. A pregnant female should not use any medication without consulting your doctor.

Set up Rewards for Every Milestone

You should reward yourself during your journey and celebrate individual milestones, such as enjoy your favorite dessert after spending 24 hours without smoking. You can watch a movie after one smoke-free week. A nice dinner, a movie or your favorite rewards after each success can increase your motivation.

Chapter 4: Successful Methods to Quit Smoking

There are a few successful methods that can help you to quit smoking and enjoy a healthy life with your friends and family members:

Cold Turkey to Quit Smoking

This is most popular and uncomfortable method to quit smoking because it involves setting a reduction or quit date and simply quit smoking without any gradual reduction, preparation or withdrawal. It may be the reason for mild or severe withdrawal symptoms, such as insomnia, fatigue, constipation, headache, sweating, poor concentration, coughing, depression and increase in appetite. It is extremely difficult to follow this approach because initial five days can be crazy for you. There are some important things that can help you to quit with this method:

- Smoke until your last day and start quitting on the weekends.
- Busy yourself in other activities, such as TV, music or extra sleep.
- Avoid frustration and depression with healthy activities.

- Avoid people with smoking habits and places where you may get cigarettes.
- Share your lousy feelings with your loved ones and request their help.
- Use non-alcoholic drinks near you and enjoy these things whenever you feel thirsty. Keep yourself hydrated by drinking plenty of water.
- Keep your hands busy by holding straws and keep your mouth busy with chewing gum.

Keep it in mind that you have to avoid cigarette at any cost because only a single or half cigarettes can be your failure. Make sure to involve yourself in other activities.

Gradual Reduction

It is a successful method and a lot of people get its help to get rid of smoking. You have to gradually reduce the number of cigarettes you smoke, such as reduce one cigarette regularly in a day and gradually reduce smoking hours. For instance, if you smoke a cigarette with an interval of one hour, you can increase this interval to two hours to three hours. If you are used to smoking 6 cigarettes in a day, you can smoke 5 or 5 ½ cigarettes on the second day. There are a few instructions that will help you to reduce your tobacco and nicotine dependence without withdrawal symptoms:

- Reduce consumption of tobacco on a regular basis.
- Always reduce the amount of tobacco each time.
- Break habit of your own brand and change brands of tobacco items.
- Reduce number of cigarettes regularly.
- Reduce inhalation and gasp without feelings its deep sensation.
- Prevent nicotine dependency by reducing intervals.
- Switch to lower nicotine, monoxide or tar content in tobacco items.

NRT can be helpful to reduce addiction to tobacco products and include gum, nasal spray, and inhaler in your routine.

Nicotine Replacement Therapy

You can get rid of smoking by replacing tobacco products with nicotine gums, patches, nasal spray, lollipops, inhalers and other products. NRT is safer than smoking, but you should consult your doctor before selecting one of them. A pregnant lady should be careful before using these things.

Nicotine Patches

These are small patches that can be attached to your skin and the nicotine will enter your bloodstream at a steady rate during the day. These can keep you steady during the day and these are safe to use during swimming and taking a bath. With these patches on your body, you should avoid smoking because you may suffer from the symptoms of nicotine overdose. This situation can lead you to death.

Drawbacks of Patches

Nicotine patches are expensive and irritate the particular area of your skin where you are wearing these patches.

Safety Tips to Use these Patches

- Patches come in 7 mg, 14 mg, and 21 mg doses and these may take 8 to 12 weeks.
- A new patch should be applied on the skin on every new day. You should select a new area of your skin and avoid application of patch on the same area for almost one week.
- Initially, you may experience mild burning, itching and tingling at the patch. These symptoms will be relieved in an hour.
- After removing this patch, your skin may turn red for a day or develop rashes. If there is any kind of swelling, you can consult a doctor.
- With nicotine patch, you can get rid of behavioral and emotional habits without any complication of nicotine withdrawal. You can use these patches with other behavioral and psychosomatic strategies.

- If you have skin allergies and irritations to adhesive tapes, you should avoid nicotine patches. It may cost between $3 and $5 per day.

Nicorette Gum

These gums can be used as cigarette replacement and it is available in different strengths, such as 2 mg and 4 mg in each gum. You can chew this gum to cut down your nicotine craving. It is important to strictly follow directions of suggested amounts to avoid its overdose. There are good for chain smokers or tobacco users to avoid withdrawal symptoms. If you become extremely anxious, you can use these gums for oral satisfaction.

Tips to Chew this Gum

- When you chew the first gum, chew it enough to make it soft and release nicotine. You have to chew a gum for almost 10 to 12 times. Once you get a tingling taste, stop chewing and keep a piece between your cheek and gum. You can release more nicotine by biting the fresh side.
- Nicotine will be absorbed through the membrane on the inner area of your cheek. It acts like a nicotine patch and slowly discharges nicotine into your blood.
- Once you feel tingling, you can stop chewing and repeat this process after a few seconds. Each gum may last for

30 minutes, but its taste and duration may vary from person to person.

- Nicotine may swallow with saliva and it may cause a few side effects, such as upset stomach, heartburn, hiccups, etc. You should avoid eating while you have gum in your mouth.
- The safe number of pieces to chew in a day may vary between 20 and 30, depending on the type of gum. Some people find it comfortable to chew between 9 and 12 pieces in a day.

Precautions and Side Effects

- Nicotine gum is not good for temporomandibular joint diseases and dental work.
- You may feel nausea, vomiting, irritation and lightheadedness.
- Loud heartbeat and excessive salivation.
- Belching the results of swallowing air during chewing the gum.

Nasal Spray

Nicotine is inhaled into the nose of a person with the help of a nasal spray or pump bottle. Nicotine will be absorbed into the lining of your nose and included in the bloodstream.

Sinus and nasal irritation are a common side effect of this spray and lots of people can tolerate this irritation. One bottle may contain 100 doses and you can use this spray almost five times in one hour. This spray can be helpful to quit smoking.

Working Pattern of Spray

Nasal spray maintains nicotine in the blood level of smokers. The smokers have a dependence on nicotine and in the absence of nicotine; you may suffer from withdrawal symptoms. This spray works similar to nicotine patches and helpful to quit smoking. It can be absorbed into your bloodstream at a faster rate.

Nicotine Inhaler

Nicotine inhaler is a device similar to cigarette and can be inhaled with the help of a mouthpiece. Every puff contains 10 times less nicotine than a puff of nicotine cigarette. The nicotine may absorb slowly and takes 10 to 15 minutes to absorb into your bloodstream. This inhaler works similar to nicotine gum and can be used as a replacement of cigarette.

It is good to relieve withdrawal symptoms and help you to quit smoking. You can use it as an aid in psychological and behavioral cessation. Nicotine inhalers are expensive than chewing gums, but make sure to consult your doctor before using this inhaler.

Nicotine Lozenge

Nicotine lozenge can easily dissolve in your mouth and release an accurate dose of nicotine to help smokers in the reduction of withdrawal symptoms. This medicine works even after lozenge vanishes. These can relieve cigarette cravings and you can use without a prescription. It can be ideal for those who want to control their nicotine intake. It is a practical aid and you can prefer it as a replacement of a chewing gum. You can also use electronic cigarettes to replace tobacco products and get rid of nicotine craving.

Quit Smoking Medications

There are a few quit smoking medications, such as:

Bupropion: It is also known as Zyban and help you to reduce withdraw symptoms. It is safe to use with NRT.

Varenicline: It is also known as Chantix and you can reduce nicotine withdrawal and reduce your urge to smoke. It is helpful to hinder the effects of nicotine and restrict users to enjoy the sensation of smoking if he/she starts again.

Safety Precautions:

If you are pregnant or nursing, you should consult your doctor before taking these medications.

If you are suffering from serious medical conditions or taking other medications, you have to talk to your doctor before taking these medicines.

If you are under 18 years, consult your doctor before using them.

Chapter 5: Diet Plan for the Success of Quit Smoking Efforts

Your brain is the center of mood and thoughts to control your movements. The brain is connected to heart and lungs with the help of arteries. These arteries supply oxygen and other important chemicals to the brain. When you smoke a cigarette, these chemicals are inhaled into your brain and actively work for 20 to 40 minutes. Once the nicotine effects and change the specialized receptor cells, this can change the pattern of thoughts, memory, and mood. Withdrawal of nicotine can change the mood of a smoker and the smoker feels irritable and anxious. In the absence of nicotine, the smoker becomes uncomfortable and it can affect the mood of smokers. This bad habit can block the carotid artery and cut off the blood supply to the brain. Smoking becomes the reason of oxidative stress.

If you are trying to get rid of smoking, it is important to focus on your diet. You should please your mood with healthy food instead of thinking about dieting. There are a few tips that can help you to increase the success rate of your quit smoking efforts:

Eating Habits

While you are trying to quit smoking, the food will take an important place in your life. You can substitute your hand-to-mouth craving with food. For instance, munch popcorns or a candy throughout the day. Eat seeds, nuts, grapes and berries or green vegetables to replace smoking. You can eat chopped carrots and salsa to supply vitamins and minerals to your body. Sugarless gum can be a good alternative to cigarette and tobacco. Keep it in mind that the tobacco has killed your taste buds and the food will taste different and better when you stop smoking.

Nicotine often suppresses your hunger and you will feel much hungrier after smoking cessation. It will be good to start your day with a healthy breakfast and avoid binge eating. You should eat 5 to 6 small meals instead of 2 to 3 larger meals. This can stimulate your metabolism and increase chances of weight loss.

Healthy Food to Enjoy

You may suffer from low blood sugar after smoking cessation; therefore, you can eat different types of snakes to slowly discharge sugar in your bloodstream. You can include slices of brown bread and wholemeal cereals in your diet. It will be good to enjoy wheat crackers, apricots, and low-fat yogurts. Healthy foods, such as fish, chicken, turkey, beans and nuts will release serotonin in your body.

Nicotine can improve withdrawal symptoms, such as anxiety and tension. You should increase consumption of protein in your diet, such as egg white, beans, fish, and poultry. It is essential to get rid of protein deprivation because the smoking depletes Vitamin C in your body. You should increase the consumption of citrus fruits for Vitamin C and reduce the risk of lung cancer. Orange and kiwis are good for your health. You can consume bananas and green vegetables to supply vitamin B in your body and improve your nervous system.

Beverages

You should avoid alcohol and caffeine because these may trigger your nicotine urge. Try to drink plenty of water throughout the day to flush out nicotine and toxins from your body. You can drink milk or herbal tea before going to bed because it will make you relax. Alcohol and caffeine should be strictly avoided because these will increase your nicotine cravings. You can include fresh fruit juices in your diet for better health.

Portion Control

It is important to avoid overeating because crackers and sweets can increase your weight. If you want to avoid an increase in weight, you should eat healthy snacks. Select a small plate to eat food and drink two glasses of water before eating something. You can include peanut butter and low-fat cheeses in your diet.

Chapter 6: Exercise Plan to Stop Smoking

If you feel a craving, you should run or do sit-ups or other exercises. After exercise, your body will release endorphins to improve your mood and you can restore energy. There are a few exercises that will help you to get rid of smoking:

Morning Walk

It is a simple fitness activity to walk in the morning and inhale fresh air. The fresh air will increase your satisfaction and calm your mind. You can think positive about your life and plan your goals.

Smoking Meditation

If you are thinking about smoking a cigarette, you have to be aware of the situation and take the packet of cigarette out of your pocket. Take out one cigarette slowly and tap the cigarette on the packet with an active mind. Your full attention should be on a cigarette. Pay attention to the sound of cigarette and smell the sensation of smoke. Imagine that smoke is released from your lungs, relax your body and enjoy the feelings. It will be similar to a boiling tea in a tea kettle and the smoke is reaching your lungs.

Initially, you can keep the cigarette in your mouth and light it. Inhale it with awareness and slowly enjoy the taste and smell. Slowly finish your cigarette and after a few days, avoid smoking cigarette. You can focus on the beauty of your surroundings, benefits of saving money and the future of your family. Start your future plans and think about spending extra money on different luxuries of your life. Inhale and exhale deeply while paying attention to the movements of your belly. Try to distract your mind from smoking and think about other activities.